Coriander Essential Oil

Benefits, Properties, Applications, Studies & Recipes

by Ann Sullivan

Published in USA by:

Ann Sullivan
217 N. Seacrest Blvd #9
Boynton Beach
FL 33425

© Copyright 2015

ISBN-13: ISBN-13: 978-1544757193
ISBN-10: ISBN-10: 1544757190

Table of Contents

Introduction

What are essential oils, and how might they be used for therapeutic purposes?

What are essential oils and how might they be used for therapeutic purposes?

Essential oils are ultra-potent oils extracted from plants and flowers that have been utilized in medicine for centuries. Presently, they are most commonly used to supplement pharmaceutical medication, but they can also be an effective alternative to pharmaceuticals in the event that there is no access to them. Before dismissing essential oils as a means to support the body's natural defenses against injury and illness, take a look at the historical evidence of the oils' medicinal competence in practice. The average age-old medical text will demonstrate that essential oils, herbs, and plenty of other natural ingredients have, for thousands of years, successfully enhanced immune function to meet and defeat any number of ailments and injuries. Though traditional medicine is considered "alternative" now, it was once the gold standard. Perhaps it still should be, as these natural age-tested remedies can fortify the body's defenses against everything from simple maladies, like headaches, cuts, and bruises to serious diseases, like cancer.

Essential oils are deemed "essential," because the oils are composed of the "essence" of the plant. The difference between essential oils and other oils – like olive oil or vegetable oil, for instance – is that essential oils have high volatility and reduced fixation, which results in faster evaporation, enabling their popular use in aromatherapy. Even at high temperatures, olive and vegetable oils do not evaporate.

Essential oils are especially necessary when it comes to a major natural or man-made disaster or potential viral outbreak. In these dire situations, people may not have quick access to their standard pharmaceutical supply; so essential oils, along with other alternative medicines, will be the go-to health aids in the case of social collapse, viral outbreak, or devastating natural disaster. When medical access is unavailable, alternatives to our modern-day standard are the only chance we have to keep pathogens at bay.

Most people do not realize that they already use essential oils every day. They are in perfumes, shampoos, soaps, and ointments; they are even used in furniture polish. Why are they found in so many aromatic products? Well, because essential oils are super concentrated aromatic liquids, so their scent is remarkably strong. Let us put this into perspective: to steam tea, use a few leaves of peppermint or juniper; to produce a single ounce of essential oil, five whole pounds of peppermint or juniper leaves are required. Some sources claim that to produce twelve pounds of essential oil would necessitate an acre of peppermint, juniper, or any other oil being produced en masse. Unlike vegetable oil, you do not often find concentrated therapeutic-grade essential oils sold in bulk; instead the oils are often sold in easily carried small, dark bottles, perfect for the GOOD bag (Get Out Of Dodge). That is exactly what this book is aiming to help people plan for – getting out of dodge with the most vital of essential oils intact, in particular a good supply of Coriander essential oil.

Why Coriander, you ask? Well, in order to get quickly up to speed on this most essential of oils, below we have provided a condensed synopsis of Coriander, after which we will outline in greater detail the oil's history, properties, and common therapeutic uses, so that you – the consumer – might have a better understanding of the oil's benefits and applications. We have even provided supportive remedies for pure Coriander, as well as blended recipes that incorporate the valuable oil. Chapter 3 will further detail past scientific research on Coriander essential oil.

Now, let's get down to it.

Summary: Coriander, or Coriandrum sativum, is extracted from the seeds, dhania or dry fruit of the Chinese Parsley plant. Originating in ancient China, the documented uses of Coriander in medicine include nausea, dysentery, hernias, and measles, to name a few. Coriander was also commonly used in ancient Egypt, and its properties are studied there to this day. Cairo University studied the oil's competence at reducing insulin and glucose levels, for which they found positive results, demonstrating Coriander's effectiveness in supporting the pancreas and aiding diabetic health.

Description: Coriander oil is commonly extracted through steam distillation. The seed is most often used. The oil is pale yellow in color, medium in consistency, and has a medium sweet spicy, woodsy scent.

Uses: Beyond those applications previously mentioned, additional uses for Coriander essential oil include supporting the body's natural defenses against arthritis, colic, digestive spasms, diabetes, flu, hypoglycemia, intestinal issues, migraines, nausea, pancreas, oily skin, muscle aches and stiffness, anorexia, colds, diarrhea, dyspepsia, flatulence, glucose levels, insulin levels, measles, neuralgia, rheumatism, gout, and spleen. When it comes to mood and emotion, Coriander relieves fear and suppresses addiction and cravings, including alcoholism, sugar, and overeating.

Properties: Antioxidant, antispasmodic, antibacterial, anti-inflammatory, anti-rheumatic, antiseptic, anti-allergenic, sedative, analgesic, aphrodisiac, digestive, stimulant, carminative, depurative, antifungal, and stomachic.

Application: Dilute 1:1 with a carrier oil. You can apply topically, inhale directly, diffuse or use as a dietary supplement.

Safety Precautions: Coriander has been approved by the FDA for internal consumption and so can be used as a dietary supplement. Do not use excessively.

Fun facts: Coriander is so named because the Latin name for "bed bug" is "koros." It was believed that the smell of Coriander was similar to that of the nighttime pest.

Another interesting fact about Coriander is that it was once so prized that only Egyptian royals were entitled to use it. In fact, King Tut and Rameses II were entombed with Coriander seeds. Coriander was also highly valued by the British colonists as it was amongst the first spices brought to America and cultivated in 1670.

Chapter 1:
Essential Oils for Aroma

Coriander oil offers a number of therapeutic benefits; but you may be wondering what these benefits are. In this chapter, we will take a closer look at the history of Coriander and its many uses.

Cultivation of Coriander

The fruit has a diameter anywhere from .06-.2 inches, depending on the variety of Coriander. Some Coriander plants, especially those which grow in temperate regions, produce small fruit. These fruit are most commonly used in the making of essential oils, as they turn out volatile oil content of .4-1.8%. Tropical and subtropical regions, like those in Australia and India, often produce plants with large fruit. These are routinely ground and blended for use in the spice trade, and their volatile oil content is relatively low, between .1-.4%.

When the plant's leaves dry and turn brown, the seeds are generally ripe for harvest. In order to harvest the seeds, the crop is cut and tied tightly in small groups. These bound groups are dried in the sun for 3-5 days, after which the sheaves are rolled or beaten in order to separate the seeds from the pods.

A History of Coriander

Coriander seeds are considered dry fruits, known as "dhania" in India. The spice is often used in Indian cuisine, and the pinene and linalool content influences the flavor of these seeds, which is warm, spicy, nutty, citrusy (or orange-flavored) and slightly lemony, particularly when crushed.

Traditionally used as a spice for culinary dishes, Coriander seed is particularly favored in India, where the spice is featured in curries, sambhar, rasam, and garam masala. In these dishes, the ground seed is combined with cumin and serves as a thickener. The roasted seed also serves as a snack in India, which is known as dhana dal.

Coriander seeds are sold either whole and dried or ground; however, when ground, the flavor of Coriander diminishes quickly, so it is more effectively applied freshly ground. When cooking, the seeds are often heated or roasted in a pan without oil, in order to produce a more pungent scent and flavor.

In other areas of the world, particularly in Europe, Africa, and Russia, Coriander seeds are used in pickling, in sausage making, and sometimes as a substitute for caraway in the making of rye bread. Both Cilantro leaves and Coriander seeds are used in Zuni cuisine, serving as salad and a meat condiment when ground with chile. The seeds are also combined with orange peel and used when brewing Belgian wheat beers to give the refreshment a citrusy flavor.

The leaves and seeds of this plant also provide different nutritional content. The seeds for instance, offer calcium, iron, selenium, magnesium, fiber, and manganese, while the leaves are much higher in vitamin and mineral content, especially when it comes to vitamins A, C, and K.

The historical roots of the plant are debatable. Growing in the wild across such an expansive region, stretching from southern Europe across to the Near East, pinpointing the plant's beginnings is hard put. However, one of the oldest archaeological discoveries of Coriander was in the Nahal Hemar Cave in Israel, where it was found alongside Neolithic Pre-Pottery era. Another of the oldest finds was in the tomb of Tutankhamen, where half a liter of Coriander was discovered. The plant is believed to have been cultivated in ancient Egypt, as it does not grow wild there. Similarly, ancient Greece is believed to have cultivated the plant since the second millennium BC, where according to the Pylos' Linear B tablets, the plant's oils served perfumery, while its seeds and leaves served as a spice and an herb respectively. Transported to North America by the British in 1670, Coriander was amongst the first plants to be cultivated by the early British colonists.

Chemical Components

In order to generate the essential oil from the Coriander fruit the seeds must be cold pressed. This results in the oil's key chemical components, which are primarily linalool, a-pinene, camphene, geraniol, and terpine.

Main Properties of Coriander Essential Oil

Along with the properties previously mentioned in the introduction, Coriander oil possesses antioxidant, antispasmodic, antibacterial, anti-inflammatory, anti-rheumatic, antiseptic, anti-allergenic, sedative, analgesic, aphrodisiac, digestive, stimulant, carminative, depurative, antifungal, and stomachic properties. With such a versatile range, Coriander is well equipped to fight off any pathogen in the body's path.

Coriander is composed of linalool, a-pinene, camphene, geraniol, and terpine. These components are what instill the enormously beneficial properties within

Coriander essential oil. We will outline these properties below.

Antioxidant

Anything high in antioxidants – whether fruit, beans, or essential oils – is a powerful advocate for your body. Antioxidants both protect against free radicals and repair their damage. What are free radicals? Free radicals are destructive chemicals that invade your body, produced by substances both inside and out. Some free radicals (or oxidants) form through normal bodily reactions, like inflammation, metabolism and aerobic respiration. Other free radicals form outside the body, but enter it due to exposure. These include harmful pollutants, toxins, smoking, alcohol, X-rays, and UV rays, to name a few. Although our bodies produce their own antioxidants, these often become damaged as we grow older; thus, introducing antioxidants into our bodies allows these nutrients and enzymes to assist in chemical reactions which destroy the oxidants or free radicals. Coriander essential oil is a moderate antioxidant, aiming to detox the body of free radicals that lead to disease. Click here to read a study about Coriander's antioxidant properties.

Antispasmodic

The antispasmodic properties of Coriander oil make it beneficial to such surgical processes as colonoscopy, gastroscopy, and intra-luminal-application double-contrast barium enema.

Antifungal

While bacteria and viruses are plenty evil, fungi commonly lead to the deadliest infections, whether external or internal. Your ears, throat, and nose are the most likely to become infected by fungi, the infections of which can be both excruciating and unsightly. If left untreated, fungal infections can kill, as they may spread to the brain. Coriander essential oil protects against these infections and more. Click here to read a study about Coriander's antifungal properties.

Antibacterial

Coriander's antibacterial properties make it a powerful protectant against diseases produced by bacteria, such as oral and digestive bacterial infection. What's great is that, unlike some prescription drugs, Coriander has no ill effects on bodily health, or on the healthy natural flora that exists within the stomach and intestines.

Antiseptic

The antiseptic and disinfectant properties of Coriander essential oil can be reaped topically, applied directly to wounds, or even through burning; the smoke from the oil may help destroy airborne germs. Internal use will help keep the wounds from becoming infections, while external use will support the body's natural function in inhibiting tetanus.

Anti-inflammatory

External or internal inflammation can be reduced through the use of Coriander essential oil. For instance, if you or your patient has swollen fingers from arthritis or a swollen knee from a sport's injury, oral application of Coriander essential oil may decrease irritation or redness, while also soothing the pain that accompanies inflammation.

Anti-allergenic

Combining both the anti-inflammatory and sedative properties culminates in an anti-allergenic effect against hyperactive allergies or reactions to external catalysts. As a sedative, Coriander calms the reaction and as an anti-inflammatory, the allergy's severity is relieved and reduced through an application of essential oil application following a reaction to food, insects, plants, or other substances that induce an allergic reaction. In the case of throat swelling, hives, hay fever, seasonal allergies, anaphylactic shock or other severe allergic reactions, this anti-allergenic effect is, quite literally, a life-saver.

Anti-rheumatic

Whereas the anti-inflammatory properties that Coriander possesses support the symptoms of arthritis, they do not necessarily influence the underlying cause. However, Coriander is also anti-rheumatic, which means it can be used to slow the disease progression of rheumatoid arthritis.

Sedative

As a sedative, Coriander sedates and calms by reducing anxiety, excitement, or irritability. Though sedatives, alone, do not alleviate pain, they do calm the patient, making them less stressed and more compliant.

Analgesic

Coriander's analgesic qualities make it an effective supplement for pain relief to be used in supporting relief from headache, sprains, injuries, wounds, scars, bruises, burns, and arthritis. It's a surefire aid for any muscle sprain due to sports or recovery pain from surgery.

Aphrodisiac

As an aphrodisiac, Coriander can help stimulate sexual arousal, thereby overriding impotence, frigidity, low libido, and erectile dysfunction.

Digestive

By boosting the production of absorptive enzymes, the digestibility of nutrients, and the secretion of digestive juices, Coriander essential oil aids the digestive tract significantly, which can greatly impact the body's overall health by increasing those nutrients absorbed from food.

Stomachic

As a stomachic, Coriander improves stomach function, boosts appetite, and helps to tone the stomach. The oil supports the body's natural function in controlling the stomach's bile, acid and gastric liquids.

Carminative

By supporting the reduction of excess gas buildup and/or removal of gas from the intestines, Coriander essential oil provides relief from abdominal pain, excess sweating, and uncomfortable indigestion.

Depurative

Coriander is a depurative, which means it has detoxifying and purifying effects.

Stimulant

Stimulants are often referred to as "uppers." This is because they produce mental or physical improvements or temporary enhancements of your bodily functions. For instance, you may grow more alert and awake or quicker on your feet after using a stimulant. Coriander can provide this temporary boost in mental and physical function.

Common Medicinal Uses

With a history rooted in international cuisine, Coriander was used to support the digestive system by smoothing digestive flow. Moreover, the oil's properties promote healthy cholesterol levels, while also supporting eye, oral and bone health. Below are a few more ways in which Coriander can play a role in your body's overall health.

Skin Health

Coriander aids in skin health, particularly when it comes to inflammation. This is because Coriander contains cineole and linoleic acid, which support arthritis and swelling. The chemical components of Coriander also help relieve rashes and other skin imperfections, as they serve skin as an anti-inflammatory. Moreover, the oil possesses antiseptic and antifungal properties that strengthen all skin types – oily or dry – by maintaining skin health. As a topical antiseptic, Coriander enhances your body's defenses against infections in wounds, as well as in burns and blisters. Moreover, the oil's antifungal properties will help protect against fungal infections, which can be highly contagious.

Cardiovascular Health

Cardiovascular health can be maintained through the abundance of vitamins and minerals found in Coriander essential oil, which include calcium, magnesium, potassium, and iron. The oil contains dietary fiber as well, which along with its other contents, helps to reduce bad cholesterol (LDL) and boost good cholesterol (HDL), resulting in better cardiovascular health. The oil's antioxidant properties and its ability to facilitate the dissolution of cholesterol that accumulates in arteries will also support cardiovascular issues, like heart disease or atherosclerosis.

Anemia

Low iron content results in anemia, which is why, with its high levels of iron, Coriander can support those who suffer from anemia and the health issues that the condition produces, such as heart palpitations, chronic fatigue, shortness of breath, and slow cognitive function. Healthy levels of iron in the body boost energy, strength, healthy bones, and also support organ system function.

Digestive Support

A healthy digestive tract means a healthy body, so maintaining good digestion can make a world of difference in overall wellness. Your digestive tract is between 25 and 30 feet long. If the length of it is not working properly, then there's a chance that food might get caught up along the tract and begin to rot within your body. Coriander effectively supports the digestive and gastrointestinal tracts' natural function by producing digestive juices and enzymes and inducing bile flow throughout the digestive organs. The antibacterial effects of many of Coriander's compounds, including cineole and limonene, help relieve diarrhea, while other of the oil's components, such as borneol and linalool, aid in proper liver function. Coriander also helps alleviate digestive issues like nausea, vomiting or stomach upset, while stimulating appetite, which makes it effective in combatting eating disorders, like anorexia. Click here to read a study on Coriander's effects on gastrointestinal health and follow this link to read about its effects on liver function.

Blood Pressure

Brimming with the vitamins and minerals, Coriander is particularly high in calcium, which is a good thing when it comes to blood pressure and hypertension. The oil's calcium ions interact with acetylcholine (aka, cholinergic), which is a neurotransmitter within the central nervous and peripheral nervous system. The interaction between the two helps to relieve tension in the blood vessels, thereby reducing blood pressure and heart rate, diminishing the risk of cardiovascular issues, like stroke or heart attack.

Oral Hygiene

The antiseptic and antibacterial properties of Coriander essential oil help kill bad breath bacteria, relieve mouth ulcers, and eliminate plaque. The oil maintains the mouth's overall health and cleanliness. In fact, chewing Coriander seeds was once a regular alternative to chewing gum, as it helped combat bad breath. Click here to read a study about Coriander's effects on oral hygiene.

Bone Health

Coriander is rich in calcium, a mineral that supports bone durability and regrowth, making the oil an effective source when it comes to strengthening bone health. Coriander can help decelerate the aging process of bones, combatting osteoporosis and other degenerative bone conditions.

Eye Health

High in antioxidants, in vitamins A and C, as well as in minerals like phosphorous, Coriander can protect against macular degeneration and vision conditions. The oil also helps reduce the stress placed on our eyes.

Diabetes & Blood Sugar

A number of studies have been done on Coriander's relationship to insulin and thereby, its potential application to diabetic health. What these studies have found is that Coriander helps boost the endocrine glands and the production of insulin in the pancreas, which aids diabetic management by increasing the blood's insulin level. Insulin helps regulate the right amount of sugar absorption and assimilation by the blood, thereby maintaining a steady blood sugar level and reducing the dangerous drops or spikes that those suffering from diabetes must manage. This property also stimulates proper metabolic function.

Safety Precautions & Common Applications

Safety

Certain adverse effects may evolve when using pure essential oils. Some essential oils should not be used when pregnant, for example, as they may cause miscarriage. Allergic reactions may occur, especially when applied topically. Always administer an allergy test before committing fully to topical application. When used with other medications, essential oils may react negatively. If you are on any current prescription medications or have a chronic illness, such as high blood pressure, epilepsy or liver disease, then researching the effects of essential oils against your own personal medical history will eliminate any potentially problematic issues.

Coriander has been approved by the FDA for internal consumption and can be used as a dietary supplement. If you have sensitive skin, dilute heavily and test before extensive use. Limit repeated use of Coriander, as overuse may cause stupefaction. To apply, dilute 1:1 with a carrier oil. You can administer topically, diffuse or use as a dietary supplement.

Blends

Oftentimes, essential oils are manufactured as blends of several pure oils. For instance, the Protective Blend of certain brands is a mix of cinnamon, clove, rosemary, and eucalyptus. This blend can be used to boost the immune system to help support colds, viruses and flus. The downside to blends is that the more oils added to the mix, the higher the probability your patient may react negatively to the blend if he/she is prone to allergies. There is also the possibility of phototoxicity when working with blends, particularly if they include citrus oils. Be sure to read your labels before administering.

Regardless of these possible effects, essential oils are a

viable option for supporting a number of conditions. Those looking to support or maintain their own personal health, or that of their families, should become educated on the uses of essential oils, their natural remedies and the methods of application. Only then can you begin building your kit of essential oils for survival.

Chapter 2:
Essential Oils for the Home

In this chapter, we'll offer various recipes for Coriander essential oil, both for pure Coriander applications and blends. For pure applications, we've provided the appropriate application and dosage to support specific ailments, from arthritis to stress. When it comes to blends, herbalists and aromatherapists often combine Coriander essential oil with ginger, cinnamon, bergamot, grapefruit, neroli, orange, lime, lemon, and other citrus fruits oils. We'll offer some fantastic blending options in the second half of this chapter.

Pure Applications

Acceptance

Promote acceptance - of both self and others - by diffusing or directly inhaling Coriander essential oil. You can also pour a drop into your hands, rub your palms together, cup them over your nose, and breathe deeply in and out for several minutes.

Anorexia

Coriander can serve as an appetite stimulant and so can support eating disorders, like anorexia. To administer, diffuse throughout the room or use as a flavor enhancer in cooking.

Arthritis

To combat the pain and inflammation of arthritis, dilute Coriander essential oil in a 1:1 ratio with a carrier oil and apply topically, massaging the oil into the joints. You can also simply diffuse or use the steam method. Steam two drops of the oil in a pan of water, remove the steaming pan from the stove, pour into a bowl, place a towel over your head and inhale. If you don't feel it's done its job the first time, you can reheat that same water and use it once more without adding more oil.

Athlete's Foot

Relieve athlete's foot by diluting Coriander essential oil

in a 1:1 ratio with a carrier oil and massaging the combo into your feet. You can also add two drops of Coriander to a foot bath or soak a pair of socks in warm water with two drops of Coriander and wear them for a half hour. Place one drop in shoes to rid of contact fungus and for extended support.

Bacterial Gastroenteritis

Combat bacterial gastroenteritis by placing several drops of Coriander essential oil in a veggie capsule. Take internally 1-3 times, daily.

Blackheads

Clear up blackheads by diluting Coriander essential oil in a 1:1 ratio with a carrier oil and applying topically to the affected area once, daily.

Candida

Eliminate candida by diluting Coriander essential oil in a 1:1 ratio with a carrier oil and massaging over affected area, into the soles of the feet, and over the abdomen. You can also take Coriander orally, through use in a capsule or as a food additive.

Cartilage Injury

To relieve cartilage injuries, dilute Coriander essential oil in a 1:1 ratio with a carrier oil and massage over the affected area or into the reflex points of the feet multiple times daily, until the injury clears up.

Circulation Stimulant

Boost blood circulation by diluting Coriander essential oil in a 1:1 ratio with a carrier oil, then apply topically, massaging the application over the heart.

Colds

Support the body's natural defenses against the cold according to its symptoms by diluting Coriander essential oil in a 1:1 ratio with a carrier oil, then apply topically, massaging it into sore muscles and joints, over the chest, and into the soles of the feet multiple times, daily. You can also diffuse throughout the home to support general health during cold/flu season.

Complexion

Use Coriander essential oil as a skin toner by diluting the oil in 1:5 ratios with purified water. Place the oil/water combo in a spray bottle and spritz on the face. Do not spray directly into eyes.

Cooking

You can use Coriander oil in cooking, as it's generally regarded as safe by the FDA. One drop (or less) to begin with; add more to taste. A little oil goes a long way.

Courage

To enhance courage or bravery, place a drop of Coriander essential oil into your hands, rub your palms together, cup them over your nose, and breathe deeply in and out for several minutes. Use daily for the best results.

Diabetes

Regulate blood sugar and insulin levels by diluting Coriander essential oil in a 1:1 ratio with a carrier oil and applying topically over the pancreas. You can also place several drops into a "00" capsule and ingest, or add a drop to each meal.

Diarrhea

If you're experiencing diarrhea, Coriander essential oil is the answer. Apply topically by diluting the oil in a 1:1 ratio with a carrier oil and massaging it into the abdomen in a counterclockwise motion, or place a drop of the oil in your drinking water throughout the day.

Digestive Aid

Coriander aids the digestive tract and can be taken orally or topically. Place a drop into your drinking water for internal administration or dilute the oil in a 1:1 ratio with a carrier oil and apply topically to the abdomen in a clockwise motion and into the reflex points of the feet. You can also diffuse throughout the home.

Energizing

Give yourself a boost of energy by diluting Coriander essential oil in a 1:1 ratio with a carrier oil and massaging it into the chest and neck, and into the reflex points on the hands and feet. You can also inhale directly for immediate energy.

Fatigue

Combat fatigue by diffusing Coriander essential oil, adding a few drops to your bathwater, or placing a drop of Coriander into your hands, rubbing your palms together, cupping them over your nose, and breathing deeply in and out for several minutes. You can also dilute and apply in a full body massage. The oil will increase blood circulation, which will boost energy and brain function.

Fear

To help eliminate unwarranted fear, dilute Coriander essential oil in a 1:1 ratio with a carrier oil and apply topically, massaging over the solar plexus and the heart. You can also administer aromatically, diffusing throughout the home or inhaling directly from the bottle.

Gas/Flatulence

Relieve gas by diluting Coriander essential oil in a 1:1 ratio with a carrier oil and applying to the abdomen in a clockwise rotation. You can also place a drop in a glass of water and take orally.

Flu

Support the body's natural defenses against the flu according to its symptoms by diluting Coriander essential oil in a 1:1 ratio with a carrier oil, then apply topically, massaging it into sore muscles and joints, over the stomach, and into the soles of the feet multiple times, daily. You can also diffuse throughout the home to support general health during cold/flu season.

Infection

To fight off infection, dilute Coriander essential oil in a 1:1 ratio with a carrier oil and apply topically to the affected area or to the soles of the feet. You can also diffuse throughout the room; whichever application is more appropriate to your specific infection.

Inflammation

Calm inflammation by diluting 1 or 2 drops of Coriander essential oil in a 1:1 ratio with a carrier oil, then apply topically, massaging it over the affected area towards the heart.

Hypoglycemia

If you're hypoglycemic, you can control your body's blood sugar levels by diluting Coriander essential oil in a 1:1 ratio with a carrier oil, then apply topically, massaging the oil into the soles of the feet and over the pancreas daily. You can also use Coriander in cooking for a similar effect.

Lead Poisoning

Combat lead poisoning by combining Coriander essential oil in a 1:1 ratio with a carrier oil and massaging toward the heart. You can also apply 1 drop to a glass of drinking water and take internally.

Measles

Relieve measles by diluting Coriander essential oil in a 1:1 ratio with a carrier oil, then apply topically, massaging it three times daily into the reflex points of the feet or over the affected area. You can also diffuse it throughout the room during times of illness.

Menstrual Cramps

Alleviate menstrual cramps by diluting Coriander essential oil in a 1:1 ratio with a carrier oil and applying topically. Massage into the lower abdomen and back and into the reflex points of the feet.

Migraines

Migraines can be relieved with Coriander oil, as the oil dilates stimulates circulation. Diffuse throughout the room or, for a more direct application, dilute Coriander essential oil in a 1:1 ratio with a carrier oil and apply topically over the area of pain, including the forehead, temple and back of the neck. Avoid the eyes.

Muscular Maintenance (Pain, Development & Toning)

To relieve sore muscles, dilute Coriander essential oil in a 1:1 ratio with a carrier oil and massage the solution into the affected area, toward the heart. You can use the same application to develop or tone muscles.

Nausea

Stave off or relieve nausea by applying a single drop to a piece of cloth or on the shirt collar to be inhaled when feeling nauseous. You can also diffuse or dilute Coriander essential oil in a 1:1 ratio with a carrier oil and massage the solution into the abdomen.

Nervousness

Nervousness can be calmed through diffusing or directly inhaling Coriander essential oil. You can also pour a drop into your hands, rub your palms together, cup them over your nose, and breathe deeply in and out for several minutes.

Neuralgia

Neuralgia and the pain caused by neuralgia can be alleviated by diluting Coriander essential oil in a 1:1 ratio with a carrier oil, then apply topically, massaging it over the affected area or into the reflex points of the feet once daily.

Pain

General pain can be eased by diluting Coriander essential oil in a 1:1 ratio with a carrier oil, then apply topically, massaging over the respective reflex points of the feet in relation to the area of bodily pain or directly into the affected area.

Rheumatism

To combat the pain and inflammation of rheumatism,

dilute Coriander essential oil in a 1:1 ratio with a carrier oil and apply topically, massaging the oil into the joints. You can also simply diffuse or use the steam method. Steam two drops of the oil in a pan of water, remove the steaming pan from the stove, pour into a bowl, place a towel over your head and inhale. If you don't feel it's done its job the first time, you can reheat that same water and use it once more without adding more oil.

Shock/Trauma

Relieve shock or trauma by diffusing or directly inhaling Coriander essential oil. You can also pour a drop into your hands, rub your palms together, cup them over your nose, and breathe deeply in and out for several minutes.

Stress

Combat stress by steaming two drops of Coriander essential oil in a pan of water, remove the steaming pan from the stove, pour into a bowl, place a towel over your head and inhale. If you don't feel it's done its job the first time, you can reheat that same water and use it once more without adding more oil. You can also diffuse or place a drop onto your shirt collar for portable stress relief.

Whiplash

Relieve whiplash by diluting Coriander essential oil in a 1:1 ratio with a carrier oil and massaging into the affected area twice, daily.

Blends

Appetite Stimulant

Ingredients

8 drops Clary Sage Essential Oil

6 drops Coriander Essential Oil

4 drops Black Pepper Essential oil

3 drops Ginger Essential Oil

2 drops Peppermint Essential Oil

Directions

To help stimulate appetite, diffuse throughout the home or pour the blend into your inhalant to use throughout the day. Those who have recently been ill or going through chemotherapy can boost their appetite through frequent inhalation.

Arthritic Massage Oil

Ingredients

2 drops Black Pepper Essential Oil

2 drops Ginger Essential Oil

3 drops Coriander Essential Oil

4 drops Helichrysum Essential Oil

5 drops Roman Chamomile Essential Oil

2 ounces Carrier Oil

Directions

To relieve arthritic pain, combine all ingredients in a small bowl, blending well. Apply topically, massaging the oil into the affected area. Use as needed.

Arthritic Massage Oil II

Ingredients

1 drop Black Pepper Essential Oil

1 drop Ginger Essential Oil

3 drops Rosemary Essential Oil

3 drops Coriander Essential Oil

4 drops Marjoram Essential Oil

6 drops Roman Chamomile Essential Oil

2 ounces Carrier Oil

Directions

To relieve arthritic pain, combine all ingredients in a small bowl, blending well. Apply topically, massaging the oil into the affected area. Use as needed.

De-stress Massage

Ingredients

5 drops Geranium Essential Oil

5 drops Coriander Essential Oil

5 drops Lavender Essential Oil

3 drops Sweet Orange Essential Oil

2 ounces Sweet Almond Oil

Directions

To wind down, de-stress, and combat anxiety, combine all ingredients in a small bowl or glass jar and mix well. Apply in a full-body massage.

Diabetes

Ingredients

2 drops Basil Essential Oil

3 drops Coriander Essential Oil

1 tsp Carrier Oil

Directions

Apply topically to the reflex points in the feet and to the back of the neck and under the tongue two times a day.

Energy Boosting Massage Oil

Ingredients

10 drops Lime Essential Oil

12 drops Bergamot Essential Oil

12 drops Lime Essential Oil

12 drops Ho Leaf Essential Oil

15 drops Coriander Essential Oil

175 mL Almond Carrier Oil

Directions

For an uplifting aromatherapy massage oil that stimulates energy, combine all ingredients in a small bowl or glass jar, blending well. Apply in a full-body massage.

Liver Detox

Ingredients

1 drop Lemon Essential Oil

1 drop Peppermint Essential Oil

1 drop Coriander Essential Oil

1 Tbsp. Organic Lemon Juice

2-4 ounces Purified Water

For a daily liver detoxifier, mix all ingredients in a glass until well combined. Drink every day in the morning as soon as you awaken. The detoxifier will help alleviate pain, regulate emotions, and boost energy Directions

Stress-Melting Bath Blend

Ingredients

2 drops Lavender Essential Oil

3 drops Jasmine Essential Oil

3 drops Coriander Essential Oil

Directions

To wind down, de-stress, and combat anxiety, add all ingredients to your bathwater and stir to disperse. Then inhale deeply while you soak for 20 minutes, but avoid getting water in your eyes, as it may sting.

Chapter 3:
Essential Oils for Body

Many studies have been done on essential oils to uncover and prove their therapeutic qualities. In the case of the great number of Coriander studies, many of the properties attributed to the essential oil (noted in this book and elsewhere) are quite often validated through the research from accredited universities and published by reputable scientific journals. In this chapter, we'll discuss a small portion of these studies. It's important to note that research on essential oils is constant and evolving. Keep up with any recent research, as it may turn up even further valuable uses of these miracle oils.

Study 1 – Oral Hygiene

In this study published by BMC Complementary & Alternative Medicine, the antimicrobial effects of Coriander essential oil on oral health were examined, with the following results: "Essential oils (EO) obtained from twenty medicinal and aromatic plants were evaluated for their antimicrobial activity against the oral pathogens Candida albicans, Fusobacterium nucleatum, Porphyromonas gingivalis, Streptococcus sanguis and Streptococcus mitis...most of the essential oils (EO) presented moderate to strong antimicrobial activity against the oral pathogens (MIC--Minimal Inhibitory Concentrations values between 0.007 and 1.00 mg/mL). The essential oil from Coriandrum sativum inhibited all oral species with MIC values from 0.007 to 0.250 mg/mL, and MBC/MFC (Minimal Bactericidal/Fungicidal Concentrations) from 0.015 to 0.500 mg/mL...The results of this research shows a great potential from the plants studied as new antimicrobial sources."

Historically, Coriander seeds were often chewed for oral hygienic purposes. This study examined the effects of Coriander and other essential oils on oral pathogens, both bacterial and fungal. The essential oils were tested against Candida albicans, Fusobacterium nucleatum, Porphyromonas gingivalis, Streptococcus sanguis and Streptococcus mitis. Candida albicans develops as yeast and filamentous cells and can potentially cause genital and oral infections. Fusobacterium nucleatum is an oral bacterium, which may result in periodontal disease through contributing to the development of plaque. Porphyromonas gingivalis is a Gram-negative, pathogenic bacterium that's found in the oral cavity, the colon, the respiratory tract, and the gastrointestinal tract. It forms in black colonies on blood agar and can cause collagen degradation which contributes to periodontal disease, as well as rheumatoid arthritis. Streptococcus sanguis and mitis are oral bacteria which cause cavities and tooth decay.

This study found that the minimum inhibitory concentration (MIC), the minimum fungicidal concentration (MFC), and the minimum bactericidal concentration (MBC) of Coriander essential oil was exceptionally effective against these strains, inhibiting all oral species. These results indicate that Coriander essential oil can be used as an oral antiseptic against these pathogens and likely, many more.

Reference:
http://www.ncbi.nlm.nih.gov/pubmed/25407737]

http://www.ncbi.nlm.nih.gov/pmc/articles/PMC4289052/pdf/12906_2013_Article_2068.pdf]

Study 2 – Anti-carcinogenic and Anti-mutagenic

In this study available on PubMed, the anti-carcinogenic and anti-mutagenic effects of Coriander essential oil were examined, with the following results: "The influence of essential oils from naturally occurring plant dietary items such as cardamom, celery seed, cumin seed, Coriander, ginger, nutmeg, and zanthoxylum on the activities of hepatic carcinogen-metabolizing enzymes (cytochrome P450, aryl hydrocarbon hydroxylase, and glutathione S-transferase) and acid-soluble sulfhydryl level was investigated...Our observations suggest that intake of essential oils affects the host enzymes associated with activation and detoxication of xenobiotic compounds, including chemical carcinogens and mutagens."

The study showed that Coriander essential oil and the other oils studied affected hepatic enzyme activities. Hepatic enzymes increase the number of carcinogens and toxins within the body. The EO's effects on this enzyme demonstrate that they may be beneficial when it comes to managing the levels of xenobiotic compounds in the human body. Xenobiotic compounds are foreign chemical substances which are not naturally found within the body, such as pollutants, chemical carcinogens and mutagens.

Reference:
http://www.ncbi.nlm.nih.gov/pubmed/8072879]

Study 3 – Alzheimer's Disease

In this study available on PubMed, the effects of Coriander essential oil on anxiety and depression in those suffering from Alzheimer's Disease were examined, with the following results: "The present study analyzed the possible anxiolytic, antidepressant and antioxidant proprieties of inhaled Coriander volatile oil extracted from Coriandrum sativum var. microcarpum in beta-amyloid (1-42) rat model of Alzheimer's disease...Exposure to Coriander volatile oil significantly improved these parameters, suggesting anxiolytic- and antidepressant-like effects. Moreover, Coriander volatile oil decreased catalase activity and increased glutathione level in the hippocampus. Our results suggest that multiple exposures to Coriander volatile oil can be useful as a mean to counteract anxiety, depression and oxidative stress in Alzheimer's disease conditions."

This study took a look at the anxiolytic, antidepressant and antioxidant effect of Coriander essential oil on rats with beta-amyloid (1-42), a model of Alzheimer's disease. The rats were then subjected to forced swimming tests and elevated plus-mazes in order to test the anxiolytic effects. The antioxidant activity was also assessed within the hippocampus, the area of the brain that is particularly significant when it comes to stress, as this is the area that processes prior memories, which then suppress or enhance a stress response. After application of Coriander essential oil, the rats' locomotor activity and times during the swimming and maze tests greatly improved. This demonstrates that Coriander may be effective in combatting oxidative stress, anxiety or depression in relation to Alzheimer's.

Reference:
http://www.ncbi.nlm.nih.gov/pubmed/24747275]

Study 4 – IBS

In this study published by the BMC Complementary & Alternative Medicine, the effects of Coriander essential oil on IBS were examined, with the following results: "Irritable bowel syndrome (IBS) is a common functional gastrointestinal disorder, which may result from alteration of the gastrointestinal microbiota following gastrointestinal infection, or with intestinal dysbiosis or small intestinal bacterial overgrowth. This may be treated with antibiotics, but there is concern that widespread antibiotic use might lead to antibiotic resistance. Some herbal medicines have been shown to be beneficial, but their mechanism(s) of action remain incompletely understood. To try to understand whether antibacterial properties might be involved in the efficacy of these herbal medicines, and to investigate potential new treatments for IBS, we have conducted a preliminary study in vitro to compare the antibacterial activity of the essential oils of culinary and medicinal herbs against the bacterium, Escherichia coli…Many of the essential oils had antibacterial activity in the three assays, suggesting that they would be good candidates for testing in clinical trials. The observed antibacterial activity of ethanolic extracts of Coriander, lemon balm and spearmint leaves suggests a mechanistic explanation for the efficacy of a mixture of Coriander, lemon balm and mint extracts against IBS in a published clinical trial."

IBS, or irritable bowel syndrome, can result in diarrhea or constipation, bloody stool, weight loss, bloating, discomfort, and chronic abdominal pain. The onset of this syndrome may occur after a stressful event and may be the result of abnormalities in the gut's flora, including bacterial growths, which might cause gastrointestinal inflammation and distorted function. The disease may even cause depression or anxiety caused by stress and reduced quality of life.

Escherichia coli is a Gram-negative bacterium that may contribute to IBS and can often result in serious food poisoning. The study showed that Coriander essential oil exhibited potent antibacterial activity against E. coli, more potent than rifaximin, the antibiotic tested. These results suggest that Coriander may support the gastrointestinal tract against this bacterium, which may make Coriander beneficial when it comes to managing IBS.

Reference:
http://www.ncbi.nlm.nih.gov/pubmed/24283351]

http://www.ncbi.nlm.nih.gov/pmc/articles/PMC4220539/pdf/1472-6882-13-338.pdf]

Study 5 – Antifungal Properties

In this study published by the journal, Molecules, the antifungal effects of Coriander essential were examined, with the following results: "The aims of this study were to test the antifungal activity, toxicity and chemical composition of essential oil from C. sativum L. fruits. The essential oil, obtained by hydro-distillation, was analyzed by gas chromatography/mass spectroscopy…C. sativum essential oil is active in vitro against M. canis and Candida spp. demonstrating good antifungal activity."

The study tested Coriander essential oil against several Candida strains, as well as Microsporum canis. Microsporum canis is a fungus that can cause ringworm in animals and tinea capitis in humans. Tinea capitis is a superficial fungal infection of the scalp that can sometimes include scaling, itching, inflammation, and pustules. Several Candida species were tested, including Candida albicans, which develops as yeast and filamentous cells, and can potentially cause genital and oral infections. Candida albicans also increases the probability of mortality in immunocompromised individuals (cancer or AIDS patients, for instance).

Coriander essential oil showed good antifungal activity against both the Candida strains and the Microsporum canis, which demonstrates that the oil can support a wide range of fungal infections.

Reference
http://www.ncbi.nlm.nih.gov/pubmed/22785271]

http://www.mdpi.com/1420-3049/17/7/8439]

Study 6 – Liver Support

In this study published by the Journal of Pharmacy & BioAllied Sciences, the effects of Coriander essential oil on the liver were examined, with the following results: "Coriandrum sativum (Linn.), a glabrous, aromatic, herbaceous annual plant, is well known for its use in jaundice. Essential oil, flavonoids, fatty acids, and sterols have been isolated from different parts of C. sativum…The results of this study have led to the conclusion that ethanolic extract of C. sativum possesses hepatoprotective activity which may be due to the antioxidant potential of phenolic compounds."

Hepatoxicity means liver damage, which is why hepatoprotection relates to the ability to protect against liver damage. The study revealed that essential oil from the Coriander plant was high in antioxidants and showed activity against carbon tetrachloride, a chemical found in everything from pesticides and fire extinguishers to refrigerants and cleaning agents. Carbon tetrachloride is often used in research to identify hepatoprotective agents, as it is amongst the most potent hepatotoxins.

Coriander essential oil helped to reduce the liver weight and the carbon tetrachloride activity in the animals tested. In fact, a 300 mg/kg dose of C. sativum extract completely eliminated the fatty deposit, the degeneration and necrosis (premature death of cells), which demonstrated the oil's antihepatotoxic activity, suggesting that Coriander is an effective liver support.

Reference
http://www.ncbi.nlm.nih.gov/pubmed/21966166]

http://www.ncbi.nlm.nih.gov/pmc/articles/PMC3178952/]

Chapter 4:
Essential Oils for Wellness

Where do essential oils come from?

Plants and plant species naturally produce essential oils for various reasons, one being to draw pollinator insects to them, another being to repel invading organisms (bacteria, animals). A number of chemical compounds compose each plant's essential oil, and the combination of these compounds are specific to each oil, which then instills in the oil its own unique properties. Essential oils can be harnessed from all sorts of plant components, including flowers, leaves, bark, fruit, roots, and resin. For instance, cinnamon oil is harnessed from bark, lemon oil from the peel, and lavender oil from lavender flowers. Certain plants can produce a few chemical variants of the same essential oil, which are acquired from different parts of the plant. Some of these parts produce a large amount of oil, while others produce just a smidgen. The oil's quality and potency depends upon a number of factors, including the subspecies of the plant, its soil conditions, the time of year and even the time of day you harvest it.

How are essential oils extracted?

Essential oils can be extracted from plants through various methods, including pressing, distillation, solvent and maceration. Let's take a brief look at each:

Pressing Method

Commonly used with citrus fruit, the pressing method extracts the oil through a technique which involves pushing the fruit peels through a press. Oily fruits and plants are best suited for this technique. Orange oil, for example, is extracted from orange skins through the pressing method.

Distillation Method

This technique harkens back to the days of old-timey moonshiners, as the same sort of method used to create strong liquor can be used to extract essential oils. Using a still, boiled water and plant materials will create steam which is then cooled by coils and condensed into a combination of water and oil. This combination doesn't mix, so the oil can then be extracted from it.

Solvent Method

Through a multi-step process, certain plant and flower oils can be extracted using alcohol and other solvents, which extort the essential oil from the plant materials.

Maceration Method

When a "carrier," or fixed oil or lard is mixed with the plant material and set out in the sun, over a period of time, the carrier oil is infused with the plant's essence. Heat sources, other than the sun, are often used to speed the process. Throughout the process, more plant material is added to produce a more potent oil.

How do you use essential oils?

Although some studies about the effectiveness of essential oils are conducted by small companies or even individuals, a number of them are conducted by the food and cosmetic industries. In general, the pharmaceutical industry shows next to no interest in herbal medicine, primarily because there are few options to patent such products. Being as such, the product's lack of profitability results in a lack of research funding. Regardless, the historical uses of essential oils tell us what we need to know: these oils have been effectively administered for centuries. The therapeutic qualifications of essential oils can be plotted in the survival of the human race across cultures and generations.

Another reason that studies on essential oils have not resulted in much conclusive evidence as to their overall effectiveness is because definitive results are sometimes difficult to prove, as the quality of each batch of oil can vary for a number of reasons. One is that essential oils are impossible to standardize. As mentioned above, even the slightest variance in soil conditions and the time of harvesting – as well as innumerable other factors – will produce a different product quality and potency. In addition, essential oils are often obtained from various species of the same plant; Eucalyptus radiata and Eucalyptus globulus can both be used in the making of therapeutic-grade eucalyptus oil and as a result, they may have slightly different properties and degrees of strength or effectiveness.

Just as there are a number of methods by which to extract essential oils, there are a number of methods to administer them therapeutically. The variety of chemical compounds in each essential oil means that their benefits and applications also vary across the board. Below are a few of these methods.

Topical Administration

Direct application of many essential oils works like a sponge, as skin sops up chemicals and other things (like sunlight, for instance). Topical application is best when you want to clear up an ailment on the skin's surface or in the underlying muscle tissue. When applying topically, you may either massage the oil into the skin or simply dab on the skin for therapeutic results. You might combine the essential oil with a carrier oil for topical use in order to dilute its potency. This is safer, as the oil is so concentrated. You may support your body's defenses against rash or muscle pain in this manner, but you should always test your patient for allergens before applying. Adverse effects are produced by natural chemicals as much as synthetic ones; poison ivy, for example.

To test for allergens, place a drop or two on your patient's inner forearm. If a rash develops within 12 to 24 hours, then the patient is allergic. In addition, phototoxicity – sun exposure resulting in an exacerbated burn – may be an issue when citrus oils are applied topically. So one must proceed with caution when applying essential oils using this method.

Inhalation Therapy

Commonly known as "aromatherapy", this essential oil application is effective for inner ailments, like sore throat or cold. In a steaming bowl of distilled or sterilized water, add a few drops of essential oil and with a towel over your head, bend over the bowl and inhale. The towel captures the vapors, making the technique even more effective. Essential oils can also be placed in a diffuser or potpourri throughout a room to produce somewhat diluted medicinal effects.

Ingestion

When using this method, proceed with caution. Direct ingestion of essential oils must be monitored and applied in small doses that are diluted in a tablespoon or more of any carrier oil – olive oil, for example. If you are unsure of dosage amounts, make a tea with the relevant herb instead. Although the effects of this diluted use may be weaker, this application is a better alternative than an overdose of essential oils.

What are the general benefits of using essential oils?

Replacement for Prescription Drugs

One practical benefit for using essential oils is, of course, their substitutive nature. Many believe that they can replace Rx drugs, which is the ultimate reason to educate yourself on their application and to begin stockpiling your essential oil supply. Although it is our opinion that 100% pure essential oils that carry no harmful side effects are better to support the body and its functions, we recommend that you consult your physician before replacing your prescription or over-the-counter medications.

One of the potential threats of economic or social collapse is the lack of resources, and primarily the inability to procure prescription drugs. Being as such, finding suitable alternatives should be a priority when prepping for the worst.

Their portability is also a major bonus when it comes to survival prepping. The fact that these ultra-concentrated oils take up little-to-no space makes toting them to your shelter all the simpler should the need arise. And because essential oils are highly concentrated, the application used in most procedures requires only a drop or two of oil, which means that tiny bottle will be long-lasting (example 15mL bottle contains approx. 250 drops).

Cheap, but Effective Alternative

Though money may be the last thing on your mind when it comes to prepping for a survival situation (money may even be obsolete in the event of social collapse), it is worth noting that the expense of essential oils pales in comparison to prescription drugs. In fact, whether or not you are forced to survive on essential oils due to a lack of prescription reserves, in some cases, you might consider substituting your prescriptions for these inexpensive alternatives regardless. Essential oils are a cheap, but equally effective alternative to prescription medicine.

No Expiration Date

Another benefit of essential oils is that they do not expire, neither do they have "proper storage" requirements. A number of medicines and medicinal products must be replaced every couple years, so this sets essential oils ahead of the pack when it comes to shelf life.

Versatility

Essential oils also offer great versatility. Apart from providing health benefits, essential oils can be repurposed for household and hygienic applications. For instance, if you're looking for something that might serve your dental hygiene needs in a time of crisis, thieves oil is your go-to essential oil. If you want to maintain your skin's health, frankincense and lavender will do the trick; the latter also serves as sunscreen, so you can prevent sun damage as well.

When it comes to the house or shelter, you can use essential oils to deodorize, which will come in handy in a disaster scenario where things might start to smell fishy due to lack of proper utilities and care. For example, after the 2011 tsunami and the subsequent nuclear reactor meltdown in Japan, a nurse named Risa Nakahira used essential oils to deodorize and sanitize putrid public bathrooms in overpopulated evacuation facilities. As relief workers searched for survivors, often wading through debris and decay, Nakahira also deodorized their boots and masks using essential oils. The possibilities of these natural oils are endless.

They are also versatile when it comes to the range of patients they're capable of supporting. The health of everyone from your great grandfather to your infant baby can be fortified with the aid of essential oils in the appropriate dosage. They even come in handy when supporting livestock or pets. From teething infants to dementia in the elderly, from teenagers with acne to dogs with urinary tract infections, essential oils can serve any patient with nearly any ailment.

Conclusion

Now that you know all about what Coriander essential oil can do for you – where it originates, how it's extracted, its benefits and properties, and the different methods of administration – you can use it confidently to support the body's defenses against health issues and start to assemble a kit of essential oils for survival. Essential oils can be purchased online or at your local holistic treatment store.

The various benefits of essential oils and their properties are countless. To build your own kit, first focus on acquiring the essential oils which may bear more relevance to your health issues or the potential health threats within your environment. In the event of a stressful event, for instance, Coriander essential oil will be one of your more crucial oils, due to its trauma and stress-supportive properties.

Used as a supplement or as your go-to for arthritis, migraines, or infections, the application of Coriander essential oil in medicine has survived for centuries and will survive centuries more. When it comes down to it, you don't need to rely on pharmaceuticals; essential oils, herbs, and plenty of other natural ingredients can be used to support any number of health issues, whether ailment or injury.

Essential oils are essential to your survival in the case

of viral outbreak, social collapse or natural disaster because, when the SHTF, your access to pharmaceuticals will likely either be limited or eliminated altogether. Alternatives to our modern-day standard will equate survival when no other option exists. And when it comes to a life-or-death situation, you can't let your health decline, no matter the state of the world.

DISCLAIMER AND/OR LEGAL NOTICES: Every effort has been made to accurately represent this book and it's potential. Results vary with every individual, and your results may or may not be different from those depicted. No promises, guarantees or warranties, whether stated or implied, have been made that you will produce any specific result from this book. Your efforts are individual and unique, and may vary from those shown. Your success depends on your efforts, background and motivation.

The material in this publication is provided for educational and informational purposes only and is not intended as medical advice. The information contained in this book should not be used to diagnose or treat any illness, metabolic disorder, disease or wellness problem. Always consult your physician or healthcare provider before beginning any nutrition or exercise program. Use of the programs, advice, and information contained in this book is at the sole choice and risk of the reader.